This journal belongs to

_____

So Forking Healthy

A Daily Food and Exercise Journal

Zeitgeist • New York

Copyright © 2021 by Penguin Random House LLC

All rights reserved.
Published in the United States by Zeitgeist, an imprint of Zeitgeist™,
a division of Penguin Random House LLC, New York.
penguinrandomhouse.com

Zeitgeist™ is a trademark of Penguin Random House LLC

ISBN: 9780593435540

Illustrations © Ku_suriuri/Shutterstock.com
Photography © Paperkites/Getty Images
Book design by Erin Yeung
Edited by Ada Fung

Printed in the United States of America
1 3 5 7 9 10 8 6 4 2

First Edition

Contents

Yes, You Can Do This

I don't count a #$&! calorie. But when I'm really trying to eat healthy, I write everything down. It really holds me accountable and puts me on a healthier path.

—TYRA BANKS, MODEL, TV PERSONALITY, AND ENTREPRENEUR

Welcome! Before you read any further, stop and pat yourself on the back. Just by cracking open this journal, you've taken the first step toward better health! Whether you're dieting to lose weight or you just want to make healthier food choices, this journal will help you reach your goals.

How's one little book supposed to do all that?

It's not rocket science. All you need to do is write down every bit of food you put in your mouth each day for 13 weeks. Doing this will help you to hold yourself accountable (if you don't lie!). And it'll help you be more mindful about what—and why—you eat. Writing everything down will make you stop and think about whether you can make a healthier choice, and whether you're actually hungry or if you're just bored or stressed (or both).

Get started by recording your current weight and measurements and setting your goals. Every day you'll jot down what you ate, how you moved your body, and how you took care of yourself. At the end of each week, you'll take stock of the past seven days, chart your progress, and make a plan for the next week. In 13 weeks, your new healthy habits will be rock-solid, and you'll be able to proudly record your new measurements and achievements and see the progress you've made.

So what the eff are you waiting for? Turn the page and get going!

How to Not Drive Yourself Insane

Eat clean to stay fit, have a burger to stay sane.

—GIGI HADID, MODEL

Here are some tips to keep in mind so that you're in control of your diet, rather than letting your diet control you.

Set realistic goals. Better to set small, incremental goals that you might even exceed rather than set yourself up for "failure" because you weren't able to meet the crazy-big goal you set.

Think "90 percent health freak, 10 percent Cookie Monster." Life is better, and a healthy diet is more sustainable, if you indulge now and again. So go ahead and eat the dang cupcake (sometimes).

Mind over mouth. Ahhh, emotional eating. Boredom snacking. Getting a serious case of the stress munchies. We've all been there. Next time you catch yourself reaching for a snack, ask yourself: Am I hungry? Or am I trying to self-soothe with food? What can I do instead to satisfy my emotional needs?

Don't let yourself get hangry. Eat more meals, but make them smaller. This way, you're less likely to get hangry (hungry + angry) and reach for junk food that you'll regret later.

Cut yourself some slack. Changing your eating habits is flippin' hard. You're going to slip up here and there. If you bite it, write it, but don't beat yourself up over it. Use it as motivation to make the next meal a healthier one.

How It Started

If you don't write down your starting measurements, then how will you be able to look back at the end and gloat over how well you did? Take this opportunity to track other health and fitness metrics in the Other Stats to Track section. (Sure, you could also measure your calves, but you're more creative than that!) How about the number of burpees you can do before you collapse on the floor? Or how far you can run before giving everyone who passes you the middle finger?

DATE:_____

CURRENT MEASUREMENTS

WEIGHT	
ARMS	
CHEST	
WAIST	
HIPS	
THIGHS	

OTHER STATS TO TRACK

How It Better Forking Go

Write down your goals here so that you can look back at the end and gloat over just how well you did. (Psst, remember to keep them realistic so that you'll be gloating and not moping.)

GOAL MEASUREMENTS

WEIGHT	
ARMS	
CHEST	
WAIST	
HIPS	
THIGHS	

OTHER #GOALS

Ready, Set, Track!

Usually, the first slip I make, I'm done. But . . . just recognizing when I go off track is an improvement and a step toward my new healthy lifestyle. When you don't feel guilty about going off track, it's easier to get right back on.

—SARA RUE, ACTOR

There's nothing like seeing exactly what you're eating every day written down in black and white to make you stick to the straight and narrow.

BE CONSISTENT AND 'FESS UP

Toss it. And not just the food that doesn't fit into your new healthy lifestyle. Toss out any negative thoughts you might have about not being able to stick to the diet. It all starts with believing you can do it.

Find a buddy. Sticking to a diet solo can be freaking hard! Buddy up with someone you can share healthy meal ideas with—or just grumble and moan with.

Make a game plan. Experts say that you're more likely to stick to a diet and see results if you plan ahead. Take some time on the weekend to meal plan for the coming week. Have healthy snacks on hand so that when the four o'clock hungries attack, you're not reaching for whatever junk is around you. Going out? Look up the menu and figure out what you'll eat before you go.

Don't bury your head in the sand. Yeah, it might suck to look at your journal and see that you went on a two-brownie-a-day bender for a week straight, but ignoring a problem doesn't make it go away. Acknowledge that it happened, figure out how and why things got off track, and recognize that you can and will do better tomorrow.

A SAMPLE DAY

Here's what a sample day might look like. Use the daily tracking pages as a guide—you don't have to track every iota of protein if that doesn't work for you, nor do you have to eat two snacks and a dessert every day. Feel free to cross things out and write in other metrics you'd rather be tracking.

DAY 1

DATE: June 18, 2021   WEIGHT: 165 lbs

TODAY'S GOAL

Take the stairs instead of the elevator

WHAT I ATE		CALORIES	FAT
		CARBS	PROTEIN
BREAKFAST	½ avocado, whole-grain toast	228	14g
		19g	2g
LUNCH	4oz grilled chicken breast, 2 cups mixed greens, 1 tbsp balsamic vinaigrette	245	8g
		4g	36g
DINNER	Turkey burger with low-fat cheddar, side salad, glass of red wine	350	12g
		23g	27g
SNACK	String cheese, small apple	150	4g
		22g	8g
SNACK/ DESSERT	¼ cup almonds	206	18g
		7g	7g

HOW I MOVED MY BODY

Walked the dog for 30 minutes in the morning, took the stairs instead of the elevator, did a 30-minute cardio video after work

WELLNESS CHECK

I DRANK ___7___ [CUPS / OUNCES] OF WATER.   I SLEPT ___7___ HOURS.

I FEEL energized from getting enough sleep last night and from my evening workout.

I FORKING ROCKED THIS TODAY: ___I didn't eat any of the cupcakes that were sitting out in the break room.

A SAMPLE WEEKLY GUT CHECK

Much like with the daily logs, you should feel free to make this weekly gut check your own.

WEEK 1 GUT CHECK

DATE: June 23, 2021

Way to crush it this week!

MEASUREMENTS

WEIGHT	164 lbs	WAIST	38 in
ARMS	13 in	HIPS	42 in
CHEST	40 in	THIGHS	21 in

OTHER STATS

Avg. number of steps/day: 9,000

Number of push-ups: 12

Minutes meditated: 70

WEEKLY REFLECTION

What went well this week?

I stuck to my goal of meditating every morning for 10 minutes. I walked and ate my lunch in a park instead of driving to eat out at a restaurant. I continue to resist the free sodas in the office.

What didn't go so hot?

I got fast food for dinner and skipped exercising on Tuesday because I was having a bad day.

What are your goals for next week?

Continue meditating for 10 minutes every morning. try a new dance cardio class with friends on Wednesday.

I'm not losing weight, I'm getting rid of it. I have no intention of finding it again.
–UNKNOWN

Eating crappy food isn't a reward—it's a punishment.

—DREW CAREY, ACTOR AND COMEDIAN

DAY 1

TODAY'S GOAL

WHAT I ATE		CALORIES	FAT
		CARBS	PROTEIN
BREAKFAST			
LUNCH			
DINNER			
SNACK			
SNACK/ DESSERT			

HOW I MOVED MY BODY

WELLNESS CHECK

I DRANK _____ [CUPS / OUNCES] OF WATER.   I SLEPT _____ HOURS.

I FEEL _____ .

I FORKING ROCKED THIS TODAY: _____

DAY 2

DATE: WEIGHT:

TODAY'S GOAL

WHAT I ATE		CALORIES	FAT
		CARBS	PROTEIN
BREAKFAST			
LUNCH			
DINNER			
SNACK			
SNACK/ DESSERT			

HOW I MOVED MY BODY

WELLNESS CHECK

I DRANK _____ [CUPS / OUNCES] OF WATER.   I SLEPT _____ HOURS.

I FEEL _____ .

I FORKING ROCKED THIS TODAY: _____

_____ .

DAY 3

TODAY'S GOAL

_____

_____

WHAT I ATE		CALORIES	FAT
		CARBS	PROTEIN
BREAKFAST			
LUNCH			
DINNER			
SNACK			
SNACK/ DESSERT			

HOW I MOVED MY BODY

_____

_____

WELLNESS CHECK

I DRANK _____ [CUPS / OUNCES] OF WATER.   I SLEPT _____ HOURS.

I FEEL _____ .

I FORKING ROCKED THIS TODAY: _____

_____ .

DAY 4

TODAY'S GOAL

_____

_____

WHAT I ATE		CALORIES	FAT
		CARBS	PROTEIN
BREAKFAST			
LUNCH			
DINNER			
SNACK			
SNACK/ DESSERT			

HOW I MOVED MY BODY

_____

_____

WELLNESS CHECK

I DRANK _____ [CUPS / OUNCES] OF WATER.   I SLEPT _____ HOURS.

I FEEL _____ .

I FORKING ROCKED THIS TODAY: _____

_____ .

DAY 5

TODAY'S GOAL

_____

_____

WHAT I ATE		CALORIES	FAT
		CARBS	PROTEIN
BREAKFAST			
LUNCH			
DINNER			
SNACK			
SNACK/ DESSERT			

HOW I MOVED MY BODY

_____

_____

WELLNESS CHECK

I DRANK _____ [CUPS / OUNCES] OF WATER.   I SLEPT _____ HOURS.

I FEEL _____ .

I FORKING ROCKED THIS TODAY: _____

_____ .

DAY 6

TODAY'S GOAL

_____

_____

WHAT I ATE	CALORIES	FAT
	CARBS	PROTEIN
BREAKFAST		
LUNCH		
DINNER		
SNACK		
SNACK/ DESSERT		

HOW I MOVED MY BODY

_____

_____

WELLNESS CHECK

I DRANK _____ [CUPS / OUNCES] OF WATER.　　　　I SLEPT _____ HOURS.

I FEEL _____ .

I FORKING ROCKED THIS TODAY: _____

_____ .

DAY 7

DATE: _____   WEIGHT: _____

TODAY'S GOAL

_____

_____

WHAT I ATE		CALORIES	FAT
		CARBS	PROTEIN
BREAKFAST			
LUNCH			
DINNER			
SNACK			
SNACK/ DESSERT			

HOW I MOVED MY BODY

_____

_____

WELLNESS CHECK

I DRANK _____ [CUPS / OUNCES] OF WATER.   I SLEPT _____ HOURS.

I FEEL _____ .

I FORKING ROCKED THIS TODAY: _____

_____ .

WEEK 1 GUT CHECK

DATE:

Way to crush it this week!

MEASUREMENTS

WEIGHT		WAIST	
ARMS		HIPS	
CHEST		THIGHS	

OTHER STATS

_____   _____

_____   _____

_____   _____

WEEKLY REFLECTION

What went well this week?

_____

_____

What didn't go so hot?

_____

_____

What are your goals for next week?

_____

_____

I'm not losing weight, I'm getting rid of it. I have no intention of finding it again.
–UNKNOWN

DAY 8

DATE: _____   WEIGHT: _____

TODAY'S GOAL

_____

_____

WHAT I ATE		CALORIES	FAT
		CARBS	PROTEIN
BREAKFAST			
LUNCH			
DINNER			
SNACK			
SNACK/ DESSERT			

HOW I MOVED MY BODY

_____

_____

WELLNESS CHECK

I DRANK _____ [CUPS / OUNCES] OF WATER.   I SLEPT _____ HOURS.

I FEEL _____ .

I FORKING ROCKED THIS TODAY: _____

_____ .

23

DAY 9

DATE: _____   WEIGHT: _____

TODAY'S GOAL

_____

_____

WHAT I ATE		CALORIES	FAT
		CARBS	PROTEIN
BREAKFAST			
LUNCH			
DINNER			
SNACK			
SNACK/ DESSERT			

HOW I MOVED MY BODY

_____

_____

WELLNESS CHECK

I DRANK _____ [CUPS / OUNCES] OF WATER.   I SLEPT _____ HOURS.

I FEEL _____ .

I FORKING ROCKED THIS TODAY: _____

_____ .

24

DAY 10

DATE: WEIGHT:

TODAY'S GOAL

_____

_____

WHAT I ATE		CALORIES	FAT
		CARBS	PROTEIN
BREAKFAST			
LUNCH			
DINNER			
SNACK			
SNACK/ DESSERT			

HOW I MOVED MY BODY

_____

_____

WELLNESS CHECK

I DRANK _____ [CUPS / OUNCES] OF WATER.   I SLEPT _____ HOURS.

I FEEL _____ .

I FORKING ROCKED THIS TODAY: _____

_____ .

DAY 11

DATE: WEIGHT:

TODAY'S GOAL

_____

_____

WHAT I ATE		CALORIES	FAT
		CARBS	PROTEIN
BREAKFAST			
LUNCH			
DINNER			
SNACK			
SNACK/ DESSERT			

HOW I MOVED MY BODY

_____

_____

WELLNESS CHECK

I DRANK _____ [CUPS / OUNCES] OF WATER.   I SLEPT _____ HOURS.

I FEEL _____ .

I FORKING ROCKED THIS TODAY: _____

_____ .

DAY 12

DATE: WEIGHT:

TODAY'S GOAL

_____

_____

WHAT I ATE		CALORIES	FAT
		CARBS	PROTEIN
BREAKFAST			
LUNCH			
DINNER			
SNACK			
SNACK/ DESSERT			

HOW I MOVED MY BODY

_____

_____

WELLNESS CHECK

I DRANK _____ [CUPS / OUNCES] OF WATER.   I SLEPT _____ HOURS.

I FEEL _____ .

I FORKING ROCKED THIS TODAY: _____

_____ .

DAY 13

TODAY'S GOAL

WHAT I ATE		CALORIES	FAT
		CARBS	PROTEIN
BREAKFAST			
LUNCH			
DINNER			
SNACK			
SNACK/ DESSERT			

HOW I MOVED MY BODY

WELLNESS CHECK

I DRANK _____ [CUPS / OUNCES] OF WATER.   I SLEPT _____ HOURS.

I FEEL _____ .

I FORKING ROCKED THIS TODAY: _____

_____ .

DAY 14

TODAY'S GOAL

_____

_____

WHAT I ATE		CALORIES	FAT
		CARBS	PROTEIN
BREAKFAST			
LUNCH			
DINNER			
SNACK			
SNACK/ DESSERT			

HOW I MOVED MY BODY

_____

_____

WELLNESS CHECK

I DRANK _____ [CUPS / OUNCES] OF WATER.   I SLEPT _____ HOURS.

I FEEL _____ .

I FORKING ROCKED THIS TODAY: _____

_____ .

WEEK 2 GUT CHECK

DATE:

Way to crush it this week!

MEASUREMENTS

WEIGHT		WAIST	
ARMS		HIPS	
CHEST		THIGHS	

OTHER STATS

_____   _____

_____   _____

_____   _____

WEEKLY REFLECTION

What went well this week?

_____

_____

What didn't go so hot?

_____

_____

What are your goals for next week?

_____

_____

Albert Einstein . . . discovered that a tiny amount of mass is equal to a huge amount of energy, which explains why, as Einstein himself so eloquently put it in a famous 1939 speech to the Physics Department at Princeton, "You have to exercise for a week to work off the thigh fat from a single Snickers."
—DAVE BARRY, HUMOR COLUMNIST AND AUTHOR

DAY 15

TODAY'S GOAL

_____

_____

WHAT I ATE		CALORIES	FAT
		CARBS	PROTEIN
BREAKFAST			
LUNCH			
DINNER			
SNACK			
SNACK/ DESSERT			

HOW I MOVED MY BODY

_____

_____

WELLNESS CHECK

I DRANK _____ [CUPS / OUNCES] OF WATER.   I SLEPT _____ HOURS.

I FEEL _____ .

I FORKING ROCKED THIS TODAY: _____

_____ .

DAY 16

DATE: WEIGHT:

TODAY'S GOAL

WHAT I ATE		CALORIES	FAT
		CARBS	PROTEIN
BREAKFAST			
LUNCH			
DINNER			
SNACK			
SNACK/ DESSERT			

HOW I MOVED MY BODY

WELLNESS CHECK

I DRANK _____ [CUPS / OUNCES] OF WATER.   I SLEPT _____ HOURS.

I FEEL _____ .

I FORKING ROCKED THIS TODAY: _____

DAY 17

DATE: WEIGHT:

TODAY'S GOAL

WHAT I ATE		CALORIES	FAT
		CARBS	PROTEIN
BREAKFAST			
LUNCH			
DINNER			
SNACK			
SNACK/ DESSERT			

HOW I MOVED MY BODY

WELLNESS CHECK

I DRANK _____ [CUPS / OUNCES] OF WATER.   I SLEPT _____ HOURS.

I FEEL _____ .

I FORKING ROCKED THIS TODAY: _____

DAY 18

TODAY'S GOAL

WHAT I ATE		CALORIES	FAT
		CARBS	PROTEIN
BREAKFAST			
LUNCH			
DINNER			
SNACK			
SNACK/ DESSERT			

HOW I MOVED MY BODY

WELLNESS CHECK

I DRANK _____ [CUPS / OUNCES] OF WATER.   I SLEPT _____ HOURS.

I FEEL _____ .

I FORKING ROCKED THIS TODAY: _____

_____ .

DAY 19

TODAY'S GOAL

WHAT I ATE		CALORIES	FAT
		CARBS	PROTEIN
BREAKFAST			
LUNCH			
DINNER			
SNACK			
SNACK/ DESSERT			

HOW I MOVED MY BODY

WELLNESS CHECK

I DRANK _____ [CUPS / OUNCES] OF WATER.   I SLEPT _____ HOURS.

I FEEL _____ .

I FORKING ROCKED THIS TODAY: _____

DAY 20

TODAY'S GOAL

_____

_____

WHAT I ATE		CALORIES	FAT
		CARBS	PROTEIN
BREAKFAST			
LUNCH			
DINNER			
SNACK			
SNACK/ DESSERT			

HOW I MOVED MY BODY

_____

_____

WELLNESS CHECK

I DRANK _____ [CUPS / OUNCES] OF WATER.   I SLEPT _____ HOURS.

I FEEL _____ .

I FORKING ROCKED THIS TODAY: _____

_____ .

DAY 21

TODAY'S GOAL

WHAT I ATE	CALORIES	FAT
	CARBS	PROTEIN
BREAKFAST		
LUNCH		
DINNER		
SNACK		
SNACK/ DESSERT		

HOW I MOVED MY BODY

WELLNESS CHECK

I DRANK _____ [CUPS / OUNCES] OF WATER.　　　　I SLEPT _____ HOURS.

I FEEL _____ .

I FORKING ROCKED THIS TODAY: _____

WEEK 3 GUT CHECK

Way to crush it this week!

MEASUREMENTS

WEIGHT		WAIST	
ARMS		HIPS	
CHEST		THIGHS	

OTHER STATS

_____   _____

_____   _____

_____   _____

WEEKLY REFLECTION

What went well this week?

_____

_____

What didn't go so hot?

_____

_____

What are your goals for next week?

_____

_____

Working out sucks. It's miserable. You sweat and you stink, but then you're done—and you see that just taking an hour three times a week can change you so much.

–KELLY OSBOURNE, TV PERSONALITY, ACTOR, AND SINGER

DAY 22

TODAY'S GOAL

WHAT I ATE		CALORIES	FAT
		CARBS	PROTEIN
BREAKFAST			
LUNCH			
DINNER			
SNACK			
SNACK/ DESSERT			

HOW I MOVED MY BODY

WELLNESS CHECK

I DRANK _____ [CUPS / OUNCES] OF WATER.   I SLEPT _____ HOURS.

I FEEL _____ .

I FORKING ROCKED THIS TODAY: _____

_____ .

DAY 23

TODAY'S GOAL

_____

_____

WHAT I ATE		CALORIES	FAT
		CARBS	PROTEIN
BREAKFAST			
LUNCH			
DINNER			
SNACK			
SNACK/ DESSERT			

HOW I MOVED MY BODY

_____

_____

WELLNESS CHECK

I DRANK _____ [CUPS / OUNCES] OF WATER.   I SLEPT _____ HOURS.

I FEEL _____ .

I FORKING ROCKED THIS TODAY: _____

_____ .

DAY 24

DATE: WEIGHT:

TODAY'S GOAL

WHAT I ATE		CALORIES	FAT
		CARBS	PROTEIN
BREAKFAST			
LUNCH			
DINNER			
SNACK			
SNACK/ DESSERT			

HOW I MOVED MY BODY

WELLNESS CHECK

I DRANK _____ [CUPS / OUNCES] OF WATER.   I SLEPT _____ HOURS.

I FEEL _____ .

I FORKING ROCKED THIS TODAY: _____

_____ .

DAY 25

DATE: _____   WEIGHT: _____

TODAY'S GOAL

_____

_____

WHAT I ATE		CALORIES	FAT
		CARBS	PROTEIN
BREAKFAST			
LUNCH			
DINNER			
SNACK			
SNACK/ DESSERT			

HOW I MOVED MY BODY

_____

_____

WELLNESS CHECK

I DRANK _____ [CUPS / OUNCES] OF WATER.   I SLEPT _____ HOURS.

I FEEL _____ .

I FORKING ROCKED THIS TODAY: _____

_____ .

DAY 26

TODAY'S GOAL

WHAT I ATE		CALORIES	FAT
		CARBS	PROTEIN
BREAKFAST			
LUNCH			
DINNER			
SNACK			
SNACK/ DESSERT			

HOW I MOVED MY BODY

WELLNESS CHECK

I DRANK _____ [CUPS / OUNCES] OF WATER.   I SLEPT _____ HOURS.

I FEEL _____ .

I FORKING ROCKED THIS TODAY: _____

DAY 27

TODAY'S GOAL

_____

_____

WHAT I ATE		CALORIES	FAT
		CARBS	PROTEIN
BREAKFAST			
LUNCH			
DINNER			
SNACK			
SNACK/ DESSERT			

HOW I MOVED MY BODY

_____

_____

WELLNESS CHECK

I DRANK _____ [CUPS / OUNCES] OF WATER.   I SLEPT _____ HOURS.

I FEEL _____ .

I FORKING ROCKED THIS TODAY: _____

_____ .

DAY 28

TODAY'S GOAL

WHAT I ATE	CALORIES	FAT
	CARBS	PROTEIN
BREAKFAST		
LUNCH		
DINNER		
SNACK		
SNACK/ DESSERT		

HOW I MOVED MY BODY

WELLNESS CHECK

I DRANK _____ [CUPS / OUNCES] OF WATER.   I SLEPT _____ HOURS.

I FEEL _____ .

I FORKING ROCKED THIS TODAY: _____

WEEK 4 GUT CHECK

Way to crush it this week!

MEASUREMENTS

WEIGHT		WAIST	
ARMS		HIPS	
CHEST		THIGHS	

OTHER STATS

_____   _____

_____   _____

_____   _____

WEEKLY REFLECTION

What went well this week?

_____

_____

What didn't go so hot?

_____

_____

What are your goals for next week?

_____

_____

I have to exercise in the morning before my brain figures out what I'm doing.
–MARSHA DOBLE, MOTIVATIONAL SPEAKER AND EXERCISE EXPERT

DAY 29

TODAY'S GOAL

_____

_____

WHAT I ATE		CALORIES	FAT
		CARBS	PROTEIN
BREAKFAST			
LUNCH			
DINNER			
SNACK			
SNACK/ DESSERT			

HOW I MOVED MY BODY

_____

_____

WELLNESS CHECK

I DRANK _____ [CUPS / OUNCES] OF WATER.   I SLEPT _____ HOURS.

I FEEL _____ .

I FORKING ROCKED THIS TODAY: _____

_____ .

DAY 30

TODAY'S GOAL

_____

_____

WHAT I ATE		CALORIES	FAT
		CARBS	PROTEIN
BREAKFAST			
LUNCH			
DINNER			
SNACK			
SNACK/ DESSERT			

HOW I MOVED MY BODY

_____

_____

WELLNESS CHECK

I DRANK _____ [CUPS / OUNCES] OF WATER.　　　　　I SLEPT _____ HOURS.

I FEEL _____ .

I FORKING ROCKED THIS TODAY: _____

_____ .

DAY 31

TODAY'S GOAL

WHAT I ATE		CALORIES	FAT
		CARBS	PROTEIN
BREAKFAST			
LUNCH			
DINNER			
SNACK			
SNACK/ DESSERT			

HOW I MOVED MY BODY

WELLNESS CHECK

I DRANK _____ [CUPS / OUNCES] OF WATER.   I SLEPT _____ HOURS.

I FEEL _____ .

I FORKING ROCKED THIS TODAY: _____

_____ .

DAY 32

DATE: WEIGHT:

TODAY'S GOAL

WHAT I ATE	CALORIES	FAT
	CARBS	PROTEIN
BREAKFAST		
LUNCH		
DINNER		
SNACK		
SNACK/ DESSERT		

HOW I MOVED MY BODY

WELLNESS CHECK

I DRANK _____ [CUPS / OUNCES] OF WATER.   I SLEPT _____ HOURS.

I FEEL _____ .

I FORKING ROCKED THIS TODAY: _____

_____ .

DAY 33

DATE: WEIGHT:

TODAY'S GOAL

_____

_____

WHAT I ATE		CALORIES	FAT
		CARBS	PROTEIN
BREAKFAST			
LUNCH			
DINNER			
SNACK			
SNACK/ DESSERT			

HOW I MOVED MY BODY

_____

_____

WELLNESS CHECK

I DRANK _____ [CUPS / OUNCES] OF WATER.   I SLEPT _____ HOURS.

I FEEL _____.

I FORKING ROCKED THIS TODAY: _____

_____.

DAY 34

TODAY'S GOAL

WHAT I ATE		CALORIES	FAT
		CARBS	PROTEIN
BREAKFAST			
LUNCH			
DINNER			
SNACK			
SNACK/ DESSERT			

HOW I MOVED MY BODY

WELLNESS CHECK

I DRANK _____ [CUPS / OUNCES] OF WATER.   I SLEPT _____ HOURS.

I FEEL _____ .

I FORKING ROCKED THIS TODAY: _____

_____ .

DAY 35

TODAY'S GOAL

_____

_____

WHAT I ATE		CALORIES	FAT
		CARBS	PROTEIN
BREAKFAST			
LUNCH			
DINNER			
SNACK			
SNACK/ DESSERT			

HOW I MOVED MY BODY

_____

_____

WELLNESS CHECK

I DRANK _____ [CUPS / OUNCES] OF WATER.   I SLEPT _____ HOURS.

I FEEL _____ .

I FORKING ROCKED THIS TODAY: _____

_____ .

WEEK 5 GUT CHECK

DATE:

Way to crush it this week!

MEASUREMENTS

WEIGHT		WAIST	
ARMS		HIPS	
CHEST		THIGHS	

OTHER STATS

_____ _____

_____ _____

_____

WEEKLY REFLECTION

What went well this week?

_____

_____

What didn't go so hot?

_____

_____

What are your goals for next week?

_____

_____

If you want to get in shape, don't sign up for fancy diet this or Crossthat the other thing. No, the way to get in shape is to go to the gym every single day, change your clothes and take a shower. If you can do that every single day for a month, pretty soon you'll start doing something while you're there.
—SETH GODIN, AUTHOR AND ENTREPRENEUR

DAY 36

TODAY'S GOAL

WHAT I ATE		CALORIES	FAT
		CARBS	PROTEIN
BREAKFAST			
LUNCH			
DINNER			
SNACK			
SNACK/ DESSERT			

HOW I MOVED MY BODY

WELLNESS CHECK

I DRANK _____ [CUPS / OUNCES] OF WATER.   I SLEPT _____ HOURS.

I FEEL _____ .

I FORKING ROCKED THIS TODAY: _____

_____ .

DAY 37

DATE: WEIGHT:

TODAY'S GOAL

WHAT I ATE		CALORIES	FAT
		CARBS	PROTEIN
BREAKFAST			
LUNCH			
DINNER			
SNACK			
SNACK/ DESSERT			

HOW I MOVED MY BODY

WELLNESS CHECK

I DRANK _____ [CUPS / OUNCES] OF WATER.   I SLEPT _____ HOURS.

I FEEL _____ .

I FORKING ROCKED THIS TODAY: _____

_____ .

DATE: WEIGHT:

TODAY'S GOAL

WHAT I ATE		CALORIES	FAT
		CARBS	PROTEIN
BREAKFAST			
LUNCH			
DINNER			
SNACK			
SNACK/ DESSERT			

HOW I MOVED MY BODY

WELLNESS CHECK

I DRANK _____ [CUPS / OUNCES] OF WATER.   I SLEPT _____ HOURS.

I FEEL _____ .

I FORKING ROCKED THIS TODAY: _____

_____ .

DAY 39

TODAY'S GOAL

_____

_____

WHAT I ATE		CALORIES	FAT
		CARBS	PROTEIN
BREAKFAST			
LUNCH			
DINNER			
SNACK			
SNACK/ DESSERT			

HOW I MOVED MY BODY

_____

_____

WELLNESS CHECK

I DRANK _____ [CUPS / OUNCES] OF WATER.   I SLEPT _____ HOURS.

I FEEL _____ .

I FORKING ROCKED THIS TODAY: _____

_____ .

DAY 40

TODAY'S GOAL

WHAT I ATE	CALORIES	FAT
	CARBS	PROTEIN
BREAKFAST		
LUNCH		
DINNER		
SNACK		
SNACK/ DESSERT		

HOW I MOVED MY BODY

WELLNESS CHECK

I DRANK _____ [CUPS / OUNCES] OF WATER.   I SLEPT _____ HOURS.

I FEEL _____ .

I FORKING ROCKED THIS TODAY: _____

DAY 41

TODAY'S GOAL

WHAT I ATE		CALORIES	FAT
		CARBS	PROTEIN
BREAKFAST			
LUNCH			
DINNER			
SNACK			
SNACK/ DESSERT			

HOW I MOVED MY BODY

WELLNESS CHECK

I DRANK _____ [CUPS / OUNCES] OF WATER.   I SLEPT _____ HOURS.

I FEEL _____ .

I FORKING ROCKED THIS TODAY: _____

_____ .

DAY 42

DATE: WEIGHT:

TODAY'S GOAL

_____

_____

WHAT I ATE		CALORIES	FAT
		CARBS	PROTEIN
BREAKFAST			
LUNCH			
DINNER			
SNACK			
SNACK/ DESSERT			

HOW I MOVED MY BODY

_____

_____

WELLNESS CHECK

I DRANK _____ [CUPS / OUNCES] OF WATER.   I SLEPT _____ HOURS.

I FEEL _____ .

I FORKING ROCKED THIS TODAY: _____

_____ .

WEEK 6 GUT CHECK

DATE:

Way to crush it this week!

MEASUREMENTS

WEIGHT		WAIST	
ARMS		HIPS	
CHEST		THIGHS	

OTHER STATS

_____   _____
_____   _____
_____   _____

WEEKLY REFLECTION

What went well this week?

_____
_____

What didn't go so hot?

_____
_____

What are your goals for next week?

_____
_____

Just try loving yourself for 30 seconds today. Smiling at yourself in the mirror. Confidence is all mental and it's time we were kind to ourselves. Just try it, if for no other reason than the other way isn't working.

–AMY SCHUMER, COMEDIAN AND ACTOR

DAY 43

TODAY'S GOAL

WHAT I ATE		CALORIES	FAT
		CARBS	PROTEIN
BREAKFAST			
LUNCH			
DINNER			
SNACK			
SNACK/ DESSERT			

HOW I MOVED MY BODY

WELLNESS CHECK

I DRANK _____ [CUPS / OUNCES] OF WATER.   I SLEPT _____ HOURS.

I FEEL _____ .

I FORKING ROCKED THIS TODAY: _____

_____ .

DAY 44

TODAY'S GOAL

WHAT I ATE		CALORIES	FAT
		CARBS	PROTEIN
BREAKFAST			
LUNCH			
DINNER			
SNACK			
SNACK/ DESSERT			

HOW I MOVED MY BODY

WELLNESS CHECK

I DRANK _____ [CUPS / OUNCES] OF WATER.   I SLEPT _____ HOURS.

I FEEL _____ .

I FORKING ROCKED THIS TODAY: _____

_____ .

DAY 45

DATE: WEIGHT:

TODAY'S GOAL

WHAT I ATE		CALORIES	FAT
		CARBS	PROTEIN
BREAKFAST			
LUNCH			
DINNER			
SNACK			
SNACK/ DESSERT			

HOW I MOVED MY BODY

WELLNESS CHECK

I DRANK _____ [CUPS / OUNCES] OF WATER.   I SLEPT _____ HOURS.

I FEEL _____ .

I FORKING ROCKED THIS TODAY: _____

_____ .

DATE: WEIGHT:

TODAY'S GOAL

_____

_____

WHAT I ATE		CALORIES	FAT
		CARBS	PROTEIN
BREAKFAST			
LUNCH			
DINNER			
SNACK			
SNACK/ DESSERT			

HOW I MOVED MY BODY

_____

_____

WELLNESS CHECK

I DRANK _____ [CUPS / OUNCES] OF WATER.   I SLEPT _____ HOURS.

I FEEL _____ .

I FORKING ROCKED THIS TODAY: _____

_____ .

DAY 47

TODAY'S GOAL

WHAT I ATE		CALORIES	FAT
		CARBS	PROTEIN
BREAKFAST			
LUNCH			
DINNER			
SNACK			
SNACK/ DESSERT			

HOW I MOVED MY BODY

WELLNESS CHECK

I DRANK _____ [CUPS / OUNCES] OF WATER.   I SLEPT _____ HOURS.

I FEEL _____ .

I FORKING ROCKED THIS TODAY: _____

DAY 48

TODAY'S GOAL

_____

_____

WHAT I ATE		CALORIES	FAT
		CARBS	PROTEIN
BREAKFAST			
LUNCH			
DINNER			
SNACK			
SNACK/ DESSERT			

HOW I MOVED MY BODY

_____

_____

WELLNESS CHECK

I DRANK _____ [CUPS / OUNCES] OF WATER.   I SLEPT _____ HOURS.

I FEEL _____ .

I FORKING ROCKED THIS TODAY: _____

_____ .

DAY 49

TODAY'S GOAL

WHAT I ATE		CALORIES	FAT
		CARBS	PROTEIN
BREAKFAST			
LUNCH			
DINNER			
SNACK			
SNACK/ DESSERT			

HOW I MOVED MY BODY

WELLNESS CHECK

I DRANK _____ [CUPS / OUNCES] OF WATER.   I SLEPT _____ HOURS.

I FEEL _____ .

I FORKING ROCKED THIS TODAY: _____

_____ .

WEEK 7 GUT CHECK

DATE:

Way to crush it this week!

MEASUREMENTS

WEIGHT		WAIST	
ARMS		HIPS	
CHEST		THIGHS	

OTHER STATS

_____   _____

_____   _____

_____   _____

WEEKLY REFLECTION

What went well this week?

_____

_____

What didn't go so hot?

_____

_____

What are your goals for next week?

_____

_____

I work hard—that's how I succeed. That's how anyone succeeds. So why in the world did I think weight loss would be any different?

–SHONDA RHIMES, TV PRODUCER, DIRECTOR, AND WRITER

DAY 50

DATE: WEIGHT:

TODAY'S GOAL

WHAT I ATE		CALORIES	FAT
		CARBS	PROTEIN
BREAKFAST			
LUNCH			
DINNER			
SNACK			
SNACK/ DESSERT			

HOW I MOVED MY BODY

WELLNESS CHECK

I DRANK _____ [CUPS / OUNCES] OF WATER.   I SLEPT _____ HOURS.

I FEEL _____.

I FORKING ROCKED THIS TODAY: _____

_____.

DAY 51

TODAY'S GOAL

_____

_____

WHAT I ATE		CALORIES	FAT
		CARBS	PROTEIN
BREAKFAST			
LUNCH			
DINNER			
SNACK			
SNACK/ DESSERT			

HOW I MOVED MY BODY

_____

_____

WELLNESS CHECK

I DRANK _____ [CUPS / OUNCES] OF WATER.   I SLEPT _____ HOURS.

I FEEL _____ .

I FORKING ROCKED THIS TODAY: _____

_____ .

DAY 52

DATE: WEIGHT:

TODAY'S GOAL

WHAT I ATE		CALORIES	FAT
		CARBS	PROTEIN
BREAKFAST			
LUNCH			
DINNER			
SNACK			
SNACK/ DESSERT			

HOW I MOVED MY BODY

WELLNESS CHECK

I DRANK _____ [CUPS / OUNCES] OF WATER.   I SLEPT _____ HOURS.

I FEEL _____ .

I FORKING ROCKED THIS TODAY: _____

_____ .

DAY 53

TODAY'S GOAL

WHAT I ATE		CALORIES	FAT
		CARBS	PROTEIN
BREAKFAST			
LUNCH			
DINNER			
SNACK			
SNACK/ DESSERT			

HOW I MOVED MY BODY

WELLNESS CHECK

I DRANK _____ [CUPS / OUNCES] OF WATER.   I SLEPT _____ HOURS.

I FEEL _____ .

I FORKING ROCKED THIS TODAY: _____

_____ .

DAY 54

TODAY'S GOAL

WHAT I ATE		CALORIES	FAT
		CARBS	PROTEIN
BREAKFAST			
LUNCH			
DINNER			
SNACK			
SNACK/ DESSERT			

HOW I MOVED MY BODY

WELLNESS CHECK

I DRANK _____ [CUPS / OUNCES] OF WATER.   I SLEPT _____ HOURS.

I FEEL _____ .

I FORKING ROCKED THIS TODAY: _____

DAY 55

TODAY'S GOAL

WHAT I ATE		CALORIES	FAT
		CARBS	PROTEIN
BREAKFAST			
LUNCH			
DINNER			
SNACK			
SNACK/ DESSERT			

HOW I MOVED MY BODY

WELLNESS CHECK

I DRANK _____ [CUPS / OUNCES] OF WATER.   I SLEPT _____ HOURS.

I FEEL _____ .

I FORKING ROCKED THIS TODAY: _____

_____ .

DAY 56

TODAY'S GOAL

_____

_____

WHAT I ATE	CALORIES	FAT
	CARBS	PROTEIN
BREAKFAST		
LUNCH		
DINNER		
SNACK		
SNACK/ DESSERT		

HOW I MOVED MY BODY

_____

_____

WELLNESS CHECK

I DRANK _____ [CUPS / OUNCES] OF WATER.   I SLEPT _____ HOURS.

I FEEL _____ .

I FORKING ROCKED THIS TODAY: _____

_____ .

WEEK 8 GUT CHECK

DATE:

Way to crush it this week!

MEASUREMENTS

WEIGHT		WAIST	
ARMS		HIPS	
CHEST		THIGHS	

OTHER STATS

_____   _____
_____   _____
_____   _____

WEEKLY REFLECTION

What went well this week?

_____
_____

What didn't go so hot?

_____
_____

What are your goals for next week?

_____
_____

Don't blame anyone or anything for your situation or problems. When you do that, you are saying that you are powerless over your own life—which is utter crap.

–JILLIAN MICHAELS, PERSONAL TRAINER AND TV PERSONALITY

DAY 57

TODAY'S GOAL

WHAT I ATE	CALORIES	FAT
	CARBS	PROTEIN
BREAKFAST		
LUNCH		
DINNER		
SNACK		
SNACK/ DESSERT		

HOW I MOVED MY BODY

WELLNESS CHECK

I DRANK _____ [CUPS / OUNCES] OF WATER.   I SLEPT _____ HOURS.

I FEEL _____ .

I FORKING ROCKED THIS TODAY: _____

_____ .

DAY 58

DATE: WEIGHT:

TODAY'S GOAL

_____

_____

WHAT I ATE		CALORIES	FAT
		CARBS	PROTEIN
BREAKFAST			
LUNCH			
DINNER			
SNACK			
SNACK/ DESSERT			

HOW I MOVED MY BODY

_____

_____

WELLNESS CHECK

I DRANK _____ [CUPS / OUNCES] OF WATER.   I SLEPT _____ HOURS.

I FEEL _____ .

I FORKING ROCKED THIS TODAY: _____

_____ .

DAY 59

TODAY'S GOAL

WHAT I ATE	CALORIES	FAT
	CARBS	PROTEIN
BREAKFAST		
LUNCH		
DINNER		
SNACK		
SNACK/ DESSERT		

HOW I MOVED MY BODY

WELLNESS CHECK

I DRANK _____ [CUPS / OUNCES] OF WATER.   I SLEPT _____ HOURS.

I FEEL _____ .

I FORKING ROCKED THIS TODAY: _____

DAY 60

TODAY'S GOAL

WHAT I ATE		CALORIES	FAT
		CARBS	PROTEIN
BREAKFAST			
LUNCH			
DINNER			
SNACK			
SNACK/ DESSERT			

HOW I MOVED MY BODY

WELLNESS CHECK

I DRANK _____ [CUPS / OUNCES] OF WATER.   I SLEPT _____ HOURS.

I FEEL _____ .

I FORKING ROCKED THIS TODAY: _____

_____ .

DAY 61

DATE: WEIGHT:

TODAY'S GOAL

| WHAT I ATE | | CALORIES | FAT |
		CARBS	PROTEIN
BREAKFAST			
LUNCH			
DINNER			
SNACK			
SNACK/ DESSERT			

HOW I MOVED MY BODY

WELLNESS CHECK

I DRANK _____ [CUPS / OUNCES] OF WATER.   I SLEPT _____ HOURS.

I FEEL _____ .

I FORKING ROCKED THIS TODAY: _____

_____ .

DAY 62

DATE: WEIGHT:

TODAY'S GOAL

WHAT I ATE		CALORIES	FAT
		CARBS	PROTEIN
BREAKFAST			
LUNCH			
DINNER			
SNACK			
SNACK/ DESSERT			

HOW I MOVED MY BODY

WELLNESS CHECK

I DRANK _____ [CUPS / OUNCES] OF WATER.   I SLEPT _____ HOURS.

I FEEL _____ .

I FORKING ROCKED THIS TODAY: _____

_____ .

DAY 63

DATE: WEIGHT:

TODAY'S GOAL

WHAT I ATE	CALORIES	FAT
	CARBS	PROTEIN
BREAKFAST		
LUNCH		
DINNER		
SNACK		
SNACK/ DESSERT		

HOW I MOVED MY BODY

WELLNESS CHECK

I DRANK _____ [CUPS / OUNCES] OF WATER.   I SLEPT _____ HOURS.

I FEEL _____ .

I FORKING ROCKED THIS TODAY: _____

_____ .

WEEK 9 GUT CHECK

DATE:

Way to crush it this week!

MEASUREMENTS

WEIGHT		WAIST	
ARMS		HIPS	
CHEST		THIGHS	

OTHER STATS

_____   _____

_____   _____

_____   _____

WEEKLY REFLECTION

What went well this week?

_____

_____

What didn't go so hot?

_____

_____

What are your goals for next week?

_____

_____

I started physically running instead of emotionally running.

–JONAH HILL, ACTOR, ON HOW HE LOST WEIGHT

DAY 64

TODAY'S GOAL

WHAT I ATE	CALORIES	FAT
	CARBS	PROTEIN
BREAKFAST		
LUNCH		
DINNER		
SNACK		
SNACK/ DESSERT		

HOW I MOVED MY BODY

WELLNESS CHECK

I DRANK _____ [CUPS / OUNCES] OF WATER.   I SLEPT _____ HOURS.

I FEEL _____ .

I FORKING ROCKED THIS TODAY: _____

DAY 65

DATE: WEIGHT:

TODAY'S GOAL

| WHAT I ATE | CALORIES | FAT |
	CARBS	PROTEIN
BREAKFAST		
LUNCH		
DINNER		
SNACK		
SNACK/ DESSERT		

HOW I MOVED MY BODY

WELLNESS CHECK

I DRANK _____ [CUPS / OUNCES] OF WATER.   I SLEPT _____ HOURS.

I FEEL _____ .

I FORKING ROCKED THIS TODAY: _____

_____ .

DAY 66

TODAY'S GOAL

WHAT I ATE		CALORIES	FAT
		CARBS	PROTEIN
BREAKFAST			
LUNCH			
DINNER			
SNACK			
SNACK/ DESSERT			

HOW I MOVED MY BODY

WELLNESS CHECK

I DRANK _____ [CUPS / OUNCES] OF WATER.   I SLEPT _____ HOURS.

I FEEL _____ .

I FORKING ROCKED THIS TODAY: _____

_____ .

DAY 67

TODAY'S GOAL

_____

_____

WHAT I ATE		CALORIES	FAT
		CARBS	PROTEIN
BREAKFAST			
LUNCH			
DINNER			
SNACK			
SNACK/ DESSERT			

HOW I MOVED MY BODY

_____

_____

WELLNESS CHECK

I DRANK _____ [CUPS / OUNCES] OF WATER.   I SLEPT _____ HOURS.

I FEEL _____ .

I FORKING ROCKED THIS TODAY: _____

_____ .

DAY 68

DATE: WEIGHT:

TODAY'S GOAL

WHAT I ATE		CALORIES	FAT
		CARBS	PROTEIN
BREAKFAST			
LUNCH			
DINNER			
SNACK			
SNACK/ DESSERT			

HOW I MOVED MY BODY

WELLNESS CHECK

I DRANK _____ [CUPS / OUNCES] OF WATER.   I SLEPT _____ HOURS.

I FEEL _____ .

I FORKING ROCKED THIS TODAY: _____

_____ .

DAY 69

TODAY'S GOAL

WHAT I ATE		CALORIES	FAT
		CARBS	PROTEIN
BREAKFAST			
LUNCH			
DINNER			
SNACK			
SNACK/ DESSERT			

HOW I MOVED MY BODY

WELLNESS CHECK

I DRANK _____ [CUPS / OUNCES] OF WATER.   I SLEPT _____ HOURS.

I FEEL _____ .

I FORKING ROCKED THIS TODAY: _____

_____ .

DAY 70

TODAY'S GOAL

_____

_____

WHAT I ATE		CALORIES	FAT
		CARBS	PROTEIN
BREAKFAST			
LUNCH			
DINNER			
SNACK			
SNACK/ DESSERT			

HOW I MOVED MY BODY

_____

_____

WELLNESS CHECK

I DRANK _____ [CUPS / OUNCES] OF WATER.   I SLEPT _____ HOURS.

I FEEL _____ .

I FORKING ROCKED THIS TODAY: _____

_____ .

WEEK 10 GUT CHECK

Way to crush it this week!

MEASUREMENTS

WEIGHT		WAIST	
ARMS		HIPS	
CHEST		THIGHS	

OTHER STATS

_____   _____

_____   _____

_____   _____

WEEKLY REFLECTION

What went well this week?

_____

_____

What didn't go so hot?

_____

_____

What are your goals for next week?

_____

_____

Your diet is a bank account. Good food choices are good investments.
—BETHENNY FRANKEL, REALITY TV PERSONALITY, AUTHOR, AND ENTREPRENEUR

DAY 71

TODAY'S GOAL

WHAT I ATE		CALORIES	FAT
		CARBS	PROTEIN
BREAKFAST			
LUNCH			
DINNER			
SNACK			
SNACK/ DESSERT			

HOW I MOVED MY BODY

WELLNESS CHECK

I DRANK _____ [CUPS / OUNCES] OF WATER.   I SLEPT _____ HOURS.

I FEEL _____ .

I FORKING ROCKED THIS TODAY: _____

_____ .

DAY 72

TODAY'S GOAL

_____

_____

WHAT I ATE		CALORIES	FAT
		CARBS	PROTEIN
BREAKFAST			
LUNCH			
DINNER			
SNACK			
SNACK/ DESSERT			

HOW I MOVED MY BODY

_____

_____

WELLNESS CHECK

I DRANK _____ [CUPS / OUNCES] OF WATER.   I SLEPT _____ HOURS.

I FEEL _____ .

I FORKING ROCKED THIS TODAY: _____

_____ .

DAY 73

DATE: WEIGHT:

TODAY'S GOAL

_____

_____

WHAT I ATE		CALORIES	FAT
		CARBS	PROTEIN
BREAKFAST			
LUNCH			
DINNER			
SNACK			
SNACK/ DESSERT			

HOW I MOVED MY BODY

_____

_____

WELLNESS CHECK

I DRANK _____ [CUPS / OUNCES] OF WATER.   I SLEPT _____ HOURS.

I FEEL _____ .

I FORKING ROCKED THIS TODAY: _____

_____ .

DAY 74

DATE: WEIGHT:

TODAY'S GOAL

WHAT I ATE		CALORIES	FAT
		CARBS	PROTEIN
BREAKFAST			
LUNCH			
DINNER			
SNACK			
SNACK/ DESSERT			

HOW I MOVED MY BODY

WELLNESS CHECK

I DRANK _____ [CUPS / OUNCES] OF WATER.   I SLEPT _____ HOURS.

I FEEL _____ .

I FORKING ROCKED THIS TODAY: _____

_____ .

DAY 75

TODAY'S GOAL

_____

_____

WHAT I ATE		CALORIES	FAT
		CARBS	PROTEIN
BREAKFAST			
LUNCH			
DINNER			
SNACK			
SNACK/ DESSERT			

HOW I MOVED MY BODY

_____

_____

WELLNESS CHECK

I DRANK _____ [CUPS / OUNCES] OF WATER.   I SLEPT _____ HOURS.

I FEEL _____ .

I FORKING ROCKED THIS TODAY: _____

_____ .

DAY 76

DATE: WEIGHT:

TODAY'S GOAL

_____

_____

WHAT I ATE		CALORIES	FAT
		CARBS	PROTEIN
BREAKFAST			
LUNCH			
DINNER			
SNACK			
SNACK/ DESSERT			

HOW I MOVED MY BODY

_____

_____

WELLNESS CHECK

I DRANK _____ [CUPS / OUNCES] OF WATER.   I SLEPT _____ HOURS.

I FEEL _____ .

I FORKING ROCKED THIS TODAY: _____

_____ .

DATE: WEIGHT:

TODAY'S GOAL

| WHAT I ATE | CALORIES | FAT |
	CARBS	PROTEIN
BREAKFAST		
LUNCH		
DINNER		
SNACK		
SNACK/ DESSERT		

HOW I MOVED MY BODY

WELLNESS CHECK

I DRANK _____ [CUPS / OUNCES] OF WATER.   I SLEPT _____ HOURS.

I FEEL _____ .

I FORKING ROCKED THIS TODAY: _____

WEEK 11 GUT CHECK

DATE:

Way to crush it this week!

MEASUREMENTS

WEIGHT		WAIST	
ARMS		HIPS	
CHEST		THIGHS	

OTHER STATS

_____   _____

_____   _____

_____   _____

WEEKLY REFLECTION

What went well this week?

_____

_____

What didn't go so hot?

_____

_____

What are your goals for next week?

_____

_____

When I buy cookies, I just eat four and throw the rest away. But first I spray them with Raid so I won't dig them out of the garbage later. Be careful, though, because that Raid really doesn't taste that bad.

–JANETTE BARBER, COMEDIAN, TV PRODUCER, AND WRITER

DAY 78

TODAY'S GOAL

WHAT I ATE	CALORIES	FAT
	CARBS	PROTEIN
BREAKFAST		
LUNCH		
DINNER		
SNACK		
SNACK/ DESSERT		

HOW I MOVED MY BODY

WELLNESS CHECK

I DRANK _____ [CUPS / OUNCES] OF WATER.   I SLEPT _____ HOURS.

I FEEL _____ .

I FORKING ROCKED THIS TODAY: _____

_____ .

DAY 79

TODAY'S GOAL

WHAT I ATE		CALORIES	FAT
		CARBS	PROTEIN
BREAKFAST			
LUNCH			
DINNER			
SNACK			
SNACK/ DESSERT			

HOW I MOVED MY BODY

WELLNESS CHECK

I DRANK _____ [CUPS / OUNCES] OF WATER.   I SLEPT _____ HOURS.

I FEEL _____ .

I FORKING ROCKED THIS TODAY: _____

_____ .

DAY 80

TODAY'S GOAL

| WHAT I ATE | CALORIES | FAT |
	CARBS	PROTEIN
BREAKFAST		
LUNCH		
DINNER		
SNACK		
SNACK/ DESSERT		

HOW I MOVED MY BODY

WELLNESS CHECK

I DRANK _____ [CUPS / OUNCES] OF WATER.   I SLEPT _____ HOURS.

I FEEL _____ .

I FORKING ROCKED THIS TODAY: _____

DAY 81

TODAY'S GOAL

WHAT I ATE	CALORIES	FAT
	CARBS	PROTEIN
BREAKFAST		
LUNCH		
DINNER		
SNACK		
SNACK/ DESSERT		

HOW I MOVED MY BODY

WELLNESS CHECK

I DRANK _____ [CUPS / OUNCES] OF WATER.   I SLEPT _____ HOURS.

I FEEL _____ .

I FORKING ROCKED THIS TODAY: _____

_____ .

DAY 82

TODAY'S GOAL

WHAT I ATE	CALORIES	FAT
	CARBS	PROTEIN
BREAKFAST		
LUNCH		
DINNER		
SNACK		
SNACK/ DESSERT		

HOW I MOVED MY BODY

WELLNESS CHECK

I DRANK _____ [CUPS / OUNCES] OF WATER.   I SLEPT _____ HOURS.

I FEEL _____ .

I FORKING ROCKED THIS TODAY: _____

_____ .

DAY 83

TODAY'S GOAL

WHAT I ATE		CALORIES	FAT
		CARBS	PROTEIN
BREAKFAST			
LUNCH			
DINNER			
SNACK			
SNACK/ DESSERT			

HOW I MOVED MY BODY

WELLNESS CHECK

I DRANK _____ [CUPS / OUNCES] OF WATER.   I SLEPT _____ HOURS.

I FEEL _____ .

I FORKING ROCKED THIS TODAY: _____

_____ .

TODAY'S GOAL

WHAT I ATE	CALORIES	FAT
	CARBS	PROTEIN
BREAKFAST		
LUNCH		
DINNER		
SNACK		
SNACK/ DESSERT		

HOW I MOVED MY BODY

WELLNESS CHECK

I DRANK _____ [CUPS / OUNCES] OF WATER.   I SLEPT _____ HOURS.

I FEEL _____ .

I FORKING ROCKED THIS TODAY: _____

_____ .

WEEK 12 GUT CHECK

Way to crush it this week!

MEASUREMENTS

WEIGHT		WAIST	
ARMS		HIPS	
CHEST		THIGHS	

OTHER STATS

_____   _____

_____   _____

_____   _____

WEEKLY REFLECTION

What went well this week?

_____

_____

What didn't go so hot?

_____

_____

What are your goals for next week?

_____

_____

I know it sounds sappy, but it was a waste. It takes a lot of creative energy to sit on your ass and figure out what you're going to eat next. I wanted to live life better.

–JOHN GOODMAN, ACTOR, ON CHOOSING TO GET HEALTHY

DAY 85

TODAY'S GOAL

WHAT I ATE		CALORIES	FAT
		CARBS	PROTEIN
BREAKFAST			
LUNCH			
DINNER			
SNACK			
SNACK/ DESSERT			

HOW I MOVED MY BODY

WELLNESS CHECK

I DRANK _____ [CUPS / OUNCES] OF WATER.   I SLEPT _____ HOURS.

I FEEL _____ .

I FORKING ROCKED THIS TODAY: _____

DAY 86

DATE: _____   WEIGHT: _____

TODAY'S GOAL

_____

_____

WHAT I ATE		CALORIES	FAT
		CARBS	PROTEIN
BREAKFAST			
LUNCH			
DINNER			
SNACK			
SNACK/ DESSERT			

HOW I MOVED MY BODY

_____

_____

WELLNESS CHECK

I DRANK _____ [CUPS / OUNCES] OF WATER.   I SLEPT _____ HOURS.

I FEEL _____ .

I FORKING ROCKED THIS TODAY: _____

_____ .

DAY 87

TODAY'S GOAL

| WHAT I ATE | CALORIES | FAT |
	CARBS	PROTEIN
BREAKFAST		
LUNCH		
DINNER		
SNACK		
SNACK/ DESSERT		

HOW I MOVED MY BODY

WELLNESS CHECK

I DRANK _____ [CUPS / OUNCES] OF WATER.   I SLEPT _____ HOURS.

I FEEL _____ .

I FORKING ROCKED THIS TODAY: _____

_____ .

DAY 88

DATE: _____   WEIGHT: _____

TODAY'S GOAL

_____

_____

WHAT I ATE		CALORIES	FAT
		CARBS	PROTEIN
BREAKFAST			
LUNCH			
DINNER			
SNACK			
SNACK/ DESSERT			

HOW I MOVED MY BODY

_____

_____

WELLNESS CHECK

I DRANK _____ [CUPS / OUNCES] OF WATER.   I SLEPT _____ HOURS.

I FEEL _____ .

I FORKING ROCKED THIS TODAY: _____

_____ .

DAY 89

TODAY'S GOAL

WHAT I ATE	CALORIES	FAT
	CARBS	PROTEIN
BREAKFAST		
LUNCH		
DINNER		
SNACK		
SNACK/ DESSERT		

HOW I MOVED MY BODY

WELLNESS CHECK

I DRANK _____ [CUPS / OUNCES] OF WATER.　　　　I SLEPT _____ HOURS.

I FEEL ....

I FORKING ROCKED THIS TODAY: _____

....

DAY 90

TODAY'S GOAL

_____

_____

WHAT I ATE		CALORIES	FAT
		CARBS	PROTEIN
BREAKFAST			
LUNCH			
DINNER			
SNACK			
SNACK/ DESSERT			

HOW I MOVED MY BODY

_____

_____

WELLNESS CHECK

I DRANK _____ [CUPS / OUNCES] OF WATER.   I SLEPT _____ HOURS.

I FEEL _____ .

I FORKING ROCKED THIS TODAY: _____

_____ .

TODAY'S GOAL

_____

_____

WHAT I ATE	CALORIES	FAT
	CARBS	**PROTEIN**
BREAKFAST		
LUNCH		
DINNER		
SNACK		
SNACK/ DESSERT		

HOW I MOVED MY BODY

_____

_____

WELLNESS CHECK

I DRANK _____ [CUPS / OUNCES] OF WATER.   I SLEPT _____ HOURS.

I FEEL _____ .

I FORKING ROCKED THIS TODAY: _____

_____ .

WEEK 13 GUT CHECK

Way to crush it this week!

MEASUREMENTS

WEIGHT		WAIST	
ARMS		HIPS	
CHEST		THIGHS	

OTHER STATS

_____   _____

_____   _____

_____   _____

WEEKLY REFLECTION

What went well this week?

_____

_____

What didn't go so hot?

_____

_____

What are your goals for next week?

_____

_____

I try to stay as regimented as possible. But if I don't have whatever that thing is for people—that cookie, that pizza, or that manhattan I like to drink every single night—I will be miserable.

–ROB McELHENNEY, ACTOR, DIRECTOR, AND PRODUCER

When you go to the grocery store, buy more bananas than cookies.

—ELIZABETH BANKS, ACTOR, DIRECTOR, AND PRODUCER

How It Went

Congratulations! It's not easy to stick to eating healthy and tracking your food, but you've forking done it for 13 weeks straight. Go ahead—take your victory lap and see how well you've done.

DATE:_____

MEASUREMENTS

	STARTING	ENDING	DIFFERENCE
WEIGHT			
ARMS			
CHEST			
WAIST			
HIPS			
THIGHS			

OTHER STATS

	STARTING	ENDING	DIFFERENCE

OK, Now What?

You can be in the habit of being healthy, or
you can be in the habit of being unhealthy.

—PETER FACINELLI, ACTOR

You didn't think you were done, did you? 13 weeks is a great start, and you've made a ton of progress—but that's a reason to keep going, not to quit. After all, you didn't get into all this just to shed a few pounds, you did it to start building a lifelong habit of eating healthy and taking good care of your body.

HOW TO KEEP THE WHOLE SHEBANG GOING

Buy this journal again. No, this isn't just a sales ploy. Tracking your food and exercise has worked for you so far, so why not keep a good thing going? Use page 123 to set new goals, and get another food journal so you can keep tracking and holding yourself accountable in the next stage of your health journey.

Check yourself before you wreck yourself. 13 weeks down, and you're feeling great. You've figured out this whole "healthy eating" thing, you're moving your body, and you're basically a health god . . . right? Except, maybe, the number on the scale isn't going down, or maybe you've noticed you're slipping back into past unhealthy habits. Hit the pause button and check in with yourself: Are you doing everything you should? If you find yourself straying too far, go back to the basics. Start counting calories again, or double-checking your portion sizes, or whatever it is that you need to do to keep yourself honest.

Plateaus aren't setbacks. That being said, plateaus are normal. It's simply not realistic to be going balls to the wall all the freaking time. Sometimes, you'll be super motivated and smash your health goals. Other times, you might just be fine with maintaining the status quo. And even if you're trying super-duper hard and doing everything right, you will plateau—that's a normal part of the weight-loss process. The important part is to not let a plateau turn into a relapse or a setback.

Switch it up. Trying to get past a plateau? Switch it up! Maybe that means cutting down on carbs and eating more protein. Or maybe that means upping the amount of exercise you're doing. Or even trying a different kind of exercise. Whatever you decide to try, switching it up not only can help you power past a plateau, it can also stop you from getting effing bored with the same old routine.

Remember your why. Cheesy, but true. Nothing will motivate you more than remembering why you're working so dang hard to get healthy and lose weight. Whether your goal is to fit into your old jeans, or to run a 5K, or to prevent disease, write it down some-where you can see it—like in this journal! Then use it to motivate you to keep going on the days when you feel like just throwing in the towel.

Write Down Those New Goals!

START DATE: _____

END DATE: _____

MEASUREMENTS

WEIGHT	
ARMS	
CHEST	
WAIST	
HIPS	
THIGHS	

OTHER STATS

Notes

Notes

Notes

Notes

Hi there,

We hope you enjoyed using *So Forking Healthy*. If you have any questions or concerns about your book, or have received a damaged copy, please contact **customerservice@penguinrandomhouse.com**. We're here and happy to help.

Also, please consider writing a review on your favorite retailer's website to let others know what you thought of the journal!

Sincerely,
The Zeitgeist Team